HCG Diet

~

Your guidebook to losing weight, fast!

By Marianne Devinson

Table of Contents

Additionally, the information in the following pages is intended only for informational purposes and should thus be thought of as universal. As befitting its nature, it is presented without assurance regarding its prolonged validity or interim quality. Trademarks that are mentioned are done without written consent and can in no way be considered an endorsement from the trademark holder.

ISBN-13: 978-1986471367

ISBN-10: 1986471365

Introduction

Congratulations on downloading this book and thank you for doing so.

The following chapters will discuss everything that you need to know to get started on the HCG diet. If you are looking to lose weight quickly to improve your health, then the HCG diet is the best option for your needs. Dieters have been able to lose a pound or more each day without any bad side effects while on the HCG diet. It is not always the easiest diet to follow, but it is the one that will give you results quickly.

This guidebook will spend some time exploring the HCG diet. You will learn everything that is needed to successfully get started on this diet plan. We will talk about what the HCG diet is, the benefits of this diet, the different phases of going on this diet, what to do if you feel hungry on this diet, and even whether you should use the injections or the drops on this diet plan. We will end the guidebook with some easy recipes that are approved for the HCG diet as well as a diet calendar that will make the HCG diet so much easier to follow and see results.

If you are looking for an easy way to lose weight quickly and efficiently, you can't go wrong with the HCG diet. Make sure to read through this guidebook to learn more about the HCG diet so you can reach your weight loss goals today.

There are plenty of books on this subject on the market, thanks again for choosing this one! Every effort was made to ensure it is full of as much useful information as possible, please enjoy!

History of the HCG Diet

The HCG diet has had a different beginning than some of the other diet plans that you may have encountered. During the early 1950s, Dr. ATW Simeons pioneered a new theory about using HCG to help people lose extra belly fat and weight.

Human Chorionic Gonadotropin, or HCG, is comprised of 244 amino acids. It is also produced in higher amounts in the placenta of a pregnant woman, can be extracted from her urine, and has historically been used to help treat infertility in females because it is effective at inducing ovulation. In addition, men who received low doses of HCG were able to see an increase in their testosterone levels.

Dr. Simeons noticed, while treating low testosterone levels with HCG, that some of the patients began to slim down a bit and most started to lose abnormal belly fat. With the knowledge that HCG can positively affect the hypothalamus gland, he then guessed that this gland was at least partly in charge of regulating normal and abnormal fat.

Over the following ten years, Dr. Simeon experimented with specific foods and specific doses of HCG. He proved that when the right diet plan and the correct amounts of HCG were followed, both females and males were able to lose a lot of fat in a short amount of time. In fact, the amount of fat lost was much more than the individual was able to do with just exercise and diet alone.

As people began to hear about this study, many doctors and health care professionals started to travel to Rome to learn more about this diet and weight loss plan. Because of all the interest in his research, Dr. Simeons published a book in 1967 called "Pounds and Inches: a New Approach to Obesity." This was meant to help lay people and health care professionals better understand what he had found during his studies.

Throughout the years, the HCG diet, which was formed from Dr. Simeons' research, started to see a decline in popularity. This was often because many of the studies that were done on this diet in the 1970s saw different results. The varying results are attributed to the studies not following the same protocol that was used by Dr. Simeons'. In addition, Dr. Simeons was never ever to receive FDA approval for his diet plan, so this set it back again.

Then in 2007, Kevin Trudeau released a book about weight loss and dieting that had a good deal of information on the HCG diet. This started to create some more interest in the work that Dr. Simeons originally did, and many professional clinics throughout the United States started offering HCG for weight loss. As more and more people started to hear about the HCG diet, it began to be seen as the miracle weight loss that everyone was looking for.

Today, many people are still looking to the HCG diet to help them lose weight and feel better. It is still sometimes hard to get ahold of the HCG that is needed for this diet plan without going to a weight loss clinic, but many people don't believe they need medical intervention to do this. Despite some of the challenges of getting HCG, it seems like Dr. Simeons' research from the 1950s is still as prevalent, and helpful to weight loss, today.

What is the HCG Diet?

There are lots of diet and weight loss programs out there that you can choose from. Some of them promise to be the miracle cure that you need to start feeling better than ever before, but not all of them can live up to that promise. With all the options out there, it can be hard to know which one can actually provide you with the right results.

One diet plan that has shown a lot of success for people trying to lose weight and get rid of the excess body fat that they are dealing with is the HCG diet. This diet requires the follower to take a natural hormone, one that the body makes during pregnancy, to help you lose weight. In addition, the follower will need to go on a really low-calorie diet to reset their metabolism. If you stick with the low calories and take the HCG, you will be able to lose a pound each day without feeling hungry all the time.

While you are on the HCG diet, you will be limited to about 500 calories each day for a total of three to six weeks. Some people who have a lot of weight to lose may go on the diet for a little longer or may do a few different cycles of the diet to help them out. You also need to take either oral drops or shots of the HCG hormone during this time to help with weight loss.

Right now, the FDA has not approved the HCG diet or the injections that you have to take. That has not stopped many people from giving them a try and enjoying the results. The shots are not considered illegal, as long as you can find a health care provider to give them to you since HCG is approved to help with fertility issues.

When you are on the HCG diet, you will not be allowed to eat much. The diet allows you to have two main meals during the day, a lunch and a dinner. Each meal needs to include one fruit, one bread, one vegetable, and one protein. You can choose to split up the meals into snacks or have a breakfast as well, but remember that you are only allowed to have up to 500 calories each day on this diet plan.

If you go on this diet plan, you will find that the amount of effort you need to put in can be hard. 500 calories a day is not that easy, and it can be really uncomfortable to do. Considering you need to stick to the 500 calories for a few weeks, and it can even be dangerous for you. It is virtually impossible to get the nutritional needs that your body requires on that many calories. But for those who are desperate to lose weight to improve their overall health, this may be the best option to help you out.

For those who are on other special diets, such as a vegetarian or vegan diet, this one will be a little harder to follow.

The HCG diet can be hard for some people to follow. You must really restrict how much you are eating for a few months, and you must take daily injections of the HCG hormone to see results. For those who have tried everything else and aren't getting the results that they want, this may be the best option to help them get the weight to finally come off.

How Does the HCG Diet Work?

If you are interested in starting on the HCG diet, there are four different phases that you will go through. Understanding these phases will help you to better stay with the HCG diet and get the results you are looking for. The different phases that you need to follow with the HCG diet include:

Phase 1

The first phase of this diet plan is known as the loading phase. This was not originally put into the HCG diet but was added later on when Kevin Trudeau reintroduced this diet. During this two-day period, you will consume foods that are high in calories until you are satisfied. You should not overeat and stretch yourself too much, but eat until you feel satisfied and full.

The point of doing this is to help satisfy some of the food addictions and cravings that you may have during the other periods on this diet plan. It has been shown that those who do not add this phase to their diet plan before entering phase two will often have stronger cravings than those who go through the loading phase.

To do this phase, you will start taking the HCG on the first day of phase one. When it comes to the foods you want to eat, make sure to eat ones that you usually crave so you can get rid of the temptation. Also, pick out foods that are higher in calories so that you can build up the fat stores in your body ahead of time.

You can basically choose any day that you would like to start your loading phase. However, it is best to not start it close to your menstrual time. Some people also choose to go with three days of loading rather than the two days. You should pick out the amount of time that you think is best for your needs.

Phase 2

The second phase will be one of the most challenging part of the HCG diet. This is the weight loss phase, where rapid weight loss will occur at a steady rate. This part will last somewhere between three and six weeks based on how much weight you need to lose. Throughout this second phase, the dieter will take the HCG injection each day, and then they need to stay on a diet that is really low in calories. When you follow this exactly, you will see weight loss each day when you weigh-in.

So, the first thing that you will do each day when you go into phase two is to take your HCG tablets, drops, or injections. You will be able to adjust the amount of HCG that you are taking based on personal needs, but most of the time the dosage is not all that important. If you feel that you are hungry all the time on this diet, you may want to increase your dosage a bit.

During phase two, you will need to stick with a diet that is under 500 calories each day. Some individuals find that they can still lose weight while eating more than then 500 calories, but to see the best results, you will stick with that calorie allotment. The HCG hormone will help you to stick with this amount of calories without feeling deprived.

During this day, you can also implement an apple day. To do an apple day, you need to start at noon on one day and then end at noon the other day. The purpose of these days is to address the issue with water retention and can help you out if you see a stall in your weight loss. During this day, you are allowed to eat up to six apples, any kind is fine, and reduce your water intake. This will help to avoid cravings and can get you back on track.

You will need to stay in phase 2 for up to six weeks. Some people have had success going for a bit longer, and it often depends on how much weight you need to lose and how fast you would like to lose it. There is a limited success going too much over six weeks though. It is often best to do one cycle of this phase, take a break, and then come back and do another six weeks at a different time if you still need to lose weight.

Phase 3

Phase three is known as the stabilization phase of this diet. This phase will happen when the dieter has finished the second phase, and they are no longer taking the HCG hormone. This will usually last for about three weeks. During this part, you will slowly add more calories and more foods to your menu. You need to slowly add in the foods, one or two at a time, so you can get used to the food and not overdo it after the low-calorie diet.

Phase three is meant to last for about three weeks. However, if you end up gaining more than two pounds in that three-week period, there are some special steps that you need to take and you will restart the three weeks. The third phase is meant to help you get back to eating more calories, without overdoing it and eating the bad foods that you did before. You will keep in this phase until you can keep your weight stabilized for a full three weeks.

Phase 4

The final stage is the maintenance stage. Here you will work to maintain the weight loss that you saw in the other phases and keep it off for good. This phase is meant to last for the rest of your life (until you want to do another cycle). The HCG plan should help you to learn how to stick with the maintenance phase without too many problems because you will learn how to avoid sugars and unhealthy fats, to only eat when you are hungry, to learn balance, and to only eat when you are actually hungry. It is all about learning how to listen to your body. If you were successful during the other phases of the HCG diet, this one should not be too hard to keep up with.

All of the phases of the HCG diet are important to helping you see the weight loss that you are looking for. Make sure to follow each one the right way, and you are sure to see results in no time.

Benefits of the HCG Diet

Before you go on any type of diet plan, it is important to know the benefits of using it. The HCG diet can be hard to use. You have to go on a very low-calorie diet for about six weeks, sticking at 500 calories or less. And you also need to take an injection or drops of HCG every day for about eight weeks while on the diet. Maintaining both of these parts can take a lot of time and dedication, and you have to be ready to keep going with it to see the results.

The good news is that there are a lot of benefits to using the HCG diet. The first benefit is that when you are taking the HCG hormone, it helps you to not feel as hungry as before. This makes it much easier to stick to the 500 calories that are required for dramatic weight loss. If you have ever tried to limit your calories in the past, you know how difficult it can be. Thinking about reducing your calories down to 500 for the course of a few months may seem impossible. But with the help of the HCG hormone, you are not only signaling the body to burn through more fat, but you are also helping to limit the cravings and can actually feel full on such a limited calorie diet.

The major benefit that you will get from the HCG diet is that you will lose a lot of weight. Once you get into the second phase, it is possible to lose a pound or more per day. The results will depend on how much weight you have to lose in the first place. Those who are only needing to lose a few pounds will find that they don't lose as much weight. But those who have a lot of weight to lose may be able to drop more than a pound each day.

This diet plan, with the help of the HCG hormone, can also help you to have enough energy to get things done during the day. With a traditional restricted calorie diet plan, you will feel sluggish and tired all of the time. You may be able to maintain the limited calories for a bit of time, but your body will feel it, and because of you being so tired, you will want to go back to your normal eating in no time. With the help of the HCG hormone, you can keep up your stores of energy and feel great the whole time.

Of course, when you are losing weight on this diet plan, there is a whole host of other benefits that you will be able to enjoy at the same time. When you lose weight, you can help to protect your heart health, lower your cholesterol levels, reduce stress, lower blood pressure, improve your mental functioning and so much more. And this diet allows you to get these great health benefits in no time without feeling deprived.

When you are looking for a diet plan that will help you to lose weight quickly and effectively so you can get your health back on track, then the HCG diet is the right one for you.

What Can You Expect?

Every person who decides to go on the HCG diet has different expectations of what will happen. This diet plan is different than what you can find when it comes to losing weight. It has been around for some time now, but you have to rely on eating very few calories and taking injections of the HCG hormone, something that is not even recommended on other diet plans.

The first thing that you will need to get used to is taking the injections. This may be a little bit scary to some people who are getting started. These injections are relatively safe and have been used in medical settings to help treat infertility problems in females. Most people who go on the HCG diet were able to self-administer these injections in no time with limited issues. If you are really worried about taking these injections, there are other methods of taking these hormones, including drops, topical options, and more.

Sometimes people will feel that the 500 calories will be too difficult for them to deal with. This is a really limited amount of food and for those dealing with low blood sugars or other health issues, limiting yourself that much can be scary. However, thanks to the HCG hormone that you are taking, you will not feel as hungry as you would when limiting these calories on your own. In many cases, you will be able to limit your calories and feel just fine.

If you find that the calories are a bit too restrictive, there are many who have upped them a little bit to feel better. This is usually reserved for those who workout quite a bit and who need a few more nutrients in their diet plan to stay healthy. Usually, you should keep it close to the 500 calories; most people will choose to go with 600 or 700 calories instead.

The biggest change that you will see when you go on this diet plan is how quickly you can see weight and fat loss. There are quite a few factors that come into play for how much weight you will be able to lose while on this diet plan. The amount that you need to lose when you start on this diet will greatly affect your weight loss. If you have a lot of weight to lose, you will see it drop off quickly at the beginning of this diet plan. It will level off the longer you are on this diet plan. Many people claim that they can lose a pound or more each day when they are on this diet plan.

Remember that this is not a full time or permanent diet plan. Other plans allow you to stay on them at least until you lose all the weight that you need or want. However, this is not advised when you are on the HCG diet. If you have a significant amount of weight to lose, it is best to do six weeks on the HCG diet and then six weeks off and then go back and forth. This makes it a bit easier to stick to the calories and ensures that you are not going to stall out on this diet plan.

Most people find that it is safe to follow this diet plan. You should learn how to listen to your body while you are on the diet though. If you feel that you are losing weight too quickly or that your body is not able to handle this low of calories, then it may be time to add more calories or to stop the diet plan.

The HCG diet is really effective for helping you to lose a lot of weight quickly, but it is quite a bit different compared to some of the other diet plans you may have tried in the past. Understanding what will happen while you are on this diet plan can make it easier to stick with this diet plan for your weight loss success.

So, this diet is working on restricting your daily calorie intake. Now, let's do some math. But before we start we need to know that one pound of fat is worth 3,500kcal or 1kg is worth 7,700kcal.

The daily caloric needs for a woman is 2,000kcal and for a man 2,500kcal. So we can now say that, in order to lose one pound of fat we need to burn 3,500kcalories. In this diet we only eat 500kcal of the 2,000kcal we need to maintain our weight. So that's 1,500 kcal we automatically burn. So we need 2.3days to lose one pound if we eat 500kcal each day.

This is the math: 3,500/1,500= 2.33

So, in one day you will see a weight loss of 0.43 pounds (1500kcal / 3500kcal). If you lose more than this, you are burning more than 2,000 calories a day. This could be due to increased physical activity, age and metabolic rate.

Injections or Drops?

When you are ready to get started on the HCG diet, you will need to choose whether you would like to use the injections or the drops to get the hormones into your body. There are some benefits and some negatives to using each one and sometimes it will come down to what you feel the most comfortable with, how much money you have to spend, and your lifestyle. The HCG diet is hard enough so if it is easier for you to take the drops, or the idea of doing an injection each day freaks you out, then stick with the drops. There are some people who say that the only effective way to do this diet plan. But when you add the HCG hormone in with a low-calorie diet, you are sure to see the weight loss that you want.

HCG Injections

When it comes to getting HCG injections, you can only get them by prescription. If you are getting them from your local pharmacy or are going on this diet with the help of your doctor, then getting the supplies can be really easy. If not, then you will need to get ahold of your supplies online. These prescriptions can be pricey, sometimes costing more than $400 or more and you may even need to visit the doctor each week as well. Some dieters order their supplies online to save some money.

When you decide to order your HCG hormone online, make sure that you get the right amount and that you can mix the solution together on your own. Some people don't have any issues with this, but it can make others nervous so keep this in mind. You also need to worry about how safe it is to order your HCG online. Most pharmacies that offer this hormone will be reputable and offer you a good product, you always need to be careful where you are ordering your supplies from.

There are also a few side effects that come with using the HCG injections. Most of these side effects will be caused by the needle. You may find bruising, and irritation from the injection site and others find that doing the injections can be painful. If these side effects make you nervous or you feel that you will not be able to perform these injections on your own, then it may be a good idea to look into the HCG drops.

HCG Drops

You can also choose to do the drops as well. This is a good option for those that need to save some money while doing this diet plan or if you are nervous about using the needles for the injections. You can either take the drops sublingually, or you can place them beneath the tongue to help them absorb better. These drops will be mixed in your home, which is important because HCG will degrade fast and you must put them in the fridge right away. You can either get these drops from your pharmacy or doctor, or you can find them through a company online.

These drops are usually going to cost less than the injections, which makes them a really good option for most people. However, there are many people who think these drops are more of a hassle than the injections. You are not allowed to drink or eat anything for half an hour after you take the drops, and this can be a problem for some. And if these drops don't absorb the proper way, you may have trouble with hunger and eating more calories than are allowed on the HCG diet.

When it comes down to it, it often depends on your personal goals and what works the best for your needs when choosing whether to go with the injections or the drops. You can choose based on what you are comfortable with, the budget you have to spend on this diet, and how easy it is for you to get the supplies. Both can be effective, especially when combined with the very low-calorie diet, in helping you to lose a lot of weight.

When Hunger Strikes

With the HCG diet, you are severely restricting the amount of calories that you are consuming. You are only allowed to eat 500 calories during the day, and this can be hard. At some point, you will probably experience hunger while being on this diet plan. However, you should note that these hunger pains will subside after about five days into the diet, as long as you take the hormone the proper way and eat the right foods.

The hunger often subsides after this length of time because your body will start to tap into the excess fat in your body and will use those calories to give you the energy that you need. This is where the fat loss and weight loss will come in, especially once you enter the process of ketosis. You simply need to be able to get through those few days of hunger to see the amazing results.

The good news for dieters is that while they may feel more hunger during days five through seven on the HCG, they are also going to see the biggest weight loss during that time. So, while you may be a bit frustrated during this time because you are feeling so hungry, you will get the reward of losing weight each day. This can be a powerful motivator when it comes to staying on the diet plan and keeping up with it to the end.

However, ignoring those hunger pains can be a big challenge during the first week on the HCG diet. You have to keep your calories down to the 500 (or close to that) if you want a chance to actually lose the weight that is promised. There are three main steps that you can follow to make it easier to get past these hunger pains. These three steps include:

Load Properly

To some people, the loading phase may seem like it is going against your weight loss goals. Why would you spend time giving in to your cravings and eating a lot of calories when you want to lose weight? But the loading phase of the HCG diet is just as important as any other one. First, it helps to provide the body with an immediate calorie reserve, enough to help you last through days three, four, and five. It also helps you to metabolize fat better because you increased how much fat you are consuming.

During the loading phase, it is best to load up on as much fat as you can. Carbs can be fine as well, but most of your focus needs to be on the fats. This helps you to have excess supplies in your body when it is time to go on the HCG diet and can make weight loss so much easier. You can have some unhealthy fats during this time, but for those who are concerned, going with healthier fats like nuts, avocado, and salmon to help you out.

Prepare foods ahead of time

Sometimes the biggest problem with this diet is that you become tempted to eat more than you should. You get hungry and then begin snacking when you are preparing your meals. Or you find that there is nothing prepared inside the house, so you go out to eat and ruin all your hard efforts.

One way to avoid this issue is to prepare your meals ahead of time. Often, it is all about convenience when it comes to which foods we will consume on the diet. Finding out the foods that are allowed on the HCG diet and then preparing them ahead of time makes our lives easier. We will eat and stick with these foods because they are already available to eat and are more convenient than making something else or going out to eat.

Cheat properly

For the most part, you should stick with the 500 calories if you would like to see all the weight loss that is promised on this diet plan. However, for some people, the 500 calories are not going to be enough. In some cases, you may want to consider adding on a few more calories. You still need to pick out foods that are approved on the HCG diet. The best option to go with is foods that are not only allowed on the HCG diet, but ones that are full of nutrients and can really fill you up. Eat plenty of these and you are less likely to feel hungry.

There are several foods that you are allowed to use as cheat foods on the HCG diet. If you find that your calories are not enough when you stick to 500, it is fine to eat as much of these as you would like, as long as you eat slowly and don't eat them simply because you are bored. Some of the foods that you can consider as your cheating foods include:

- Green vegetables: Green vegetables are usually fine to eat extra of on the HCG diet. Just make sure that you are not eating cucumbers or anything else that has seeds inside of them because these are going to contain more carbs than other options.

- Chicken bouillon: These cubes or pouches will usually contain fewer than 30 calories each, but adding some to water and sipping can be really filling. Some people are worried about all the extra sodium. But doing this on occasion is not going to cause that much of an issue.

- Beef jerky: If you include beef jerky in your diet, make sure you are getting some of the good kind with lots of protein inside of it. Beef jerky has a good protein, fats, and carb ratio, so it is the perfect snack food. Adding a few ounces between your meals, and maybe adding in some celery stalks can help you to feel less hungry while losing weight.

There will be times when you will feel hungry on the HCG diet, mainly because you are cutting down on your calories quite a bit. The good news is that your body will soon tap into the excess stores of fat inside and you will see a great amount of fat and weight loss in no time. Add in the HCG hormone, and you will be able to see weight loss, without a lot of hunger, in no time.

Another thing that the hormone does is to make you feel like you are full.

FAQs About the HCG Diet

Getting started on the HCG diet can be difficult. You have to be careful about how many calories you are taking in each day to keep it low. You also need to take some injections or some drops if you would like to see the results. All of this needs to come together to see the weight loss that you are promised. The good news is that if you are successful with following all the steps, you can easily lose one or more pounds each day. For those who have a lot of weight to lose and have tried everything else, this may be the diet plan you need. If you are interested in the HCG diet, make sure to take a look at some of these FAQ's to help you determine if the HCG diet is the right one for you.

What is HCG

HCG, or Human Chorionic Gonadotropin, is a hormone that is already produced in women and men in small amounts. Pregnant women often produce this in higher amounts. The HCG is in charge of influencing how the metabolism works by stimulating the hypothalamus. The HCG hormone has traditionally been used in medicine to help with infertility problems in women and with low testosterone levels in men.

The idea of HCG in this diet plan is to speed up the metabolism so that you can lose weight even faster. You would take the HCG hormone either in the form of drops or an injection, to help with the weight loss. When you combine it with a very low-calorie diet, you will be able to see a lot of weight loss in a short amount of time.

Is it legal to use HCG for weight loss?

It is legal to use HCG for weight loss. The FDA does not technically endorse the 500 calorie diet that comes with the HCG diet, but it is legal to use HCG. In fact, HCG is currently used as a way to treat infertility in women and many doctors are fine with prescribing it as a weight loss tool. There are also some newer versions of the HCG diet that allow for more of a calorie allowance that are allowed by the FDA.

Who will do well with the HCG diet?

The majority of patients who are overweight, but otherwise healthy, whether they are men or women, can be considered potential patients for using the HCG diet for weight loss. It is best if you take some time to talk to your doctor before you start on this diet. This ensures that you don't have any underlying conditions that may be affected when you go on this diet plan.

Are there side effects to the drops or the injections?

There are some side effects to going on the HCG diet and using both the drops and the injections. However, very few patients ever report any of these side effects. When the HCG hormone is used to help as a fertility treatment, the larger amount that is needed for that treatment can sometimes cause pregnancy symptoms and the occasional headache.

However, it is important to note that when you are following the HCG diet, you will take a much lower dosage of HCG than is used in fertility treatments. Sometimes the patient will experience some hunger, lightheadedness, and hungry. It is often considered the fault of the protocol, and the lack of calories that you are eating, that will cause these issues.

How much can I lose on this diet plan?

The amount that you can lose on this diet plan will vary based on a number of factors. Your age, your weight, your metabolism, and whether you are a male or female can all determine how much weight you can lose when you go on the HCG diet.

There was a recent poll conducted that included more than 7000 people who have gone on the HCG diet. The results showed that on average, the participants were losing half a pound to a pound each day. There were even some participants who lost up to 3 pounds in one day. These are the average results from the diet plan, and each person will see different results when they go on the HCG diet. As long as you learn your own body chemistry so you can make changes if needed, then you will be able to lose weight with this diet plan.

Is it safe for men to take HCG?

The HCG hormone is actually found in men naturally. While you will find HCG in the highest concentrations in women who are pregnant, it is produced in a decent amount in anyone. This means that there are men who have the HCG hormone naturally as well. In fact, there are millions of men who have been about to use the HCG diet to help them lose weight without a lot of issues.

Where do I get the injections or drops?

There are several places where you can get hold of the injections or the drops. If you are working along with a healthcare professional to follow this diet, you will be able to get the HCG hormone from them. This is a good way to get the HCG hormone because you know that it will be safe and won't have to do as much research about it. If you would like to reduce the costs a bit or you are going on this diet plan without the supervision of a doctor or other healthcare professional, then you can choose to purchase the drops or the injections online and mix the solution yourself.

Is it really healthy to lose this much weight each day?

When you go on the HCG diet, you will see a lot of weight loss in a short amount of time. This diet plan is successful at giving you fast weight loss while stimulating the body to maintain the lean muscle in the long run. Since your weight loss will come right from unhealthy fats, it is not going to strip the body of the muscles that are in the body. When you add in all the healthy foods you will learn how to cook, you will still be able to lose weight (while still nourishing the body all at the same time. in the end, you will end up eating healthier when you are done than you were in the beginning.

Are the HCG injections painful?

The injections that you get of HCG to help with weight loss will be administered through a needle that is small and very fine. In addition, the HCG hormone will be administered in an area that is not that sensitive. Most dieters report that the injections are not all that painful. For those who are worried that these injections will be too painful or who may not be able to give themselves the injections, it is possible to use the drops instead.

Where do I inject the shots?

The easiest, as well as the most comfortable, place for you to inject the HCG hormone is right in the stomach. You should go about two inches from the naval. You can also administer these injections in the thigh or on the back of the arm if this is easier for you.

Will I be hungry on the HCG diet?

There are some dieters who claim that they do feel hungry when they are on this diet in the beginning. This is because they are following a very low-calorie diet to lose weight. But with the help of the HCG hormone and the fat burning that should occur on this diet plan, the hunger should not last long.

Am I going to gain all the weight back when I'm done?

Not only is the HCG diet great for helping you to lose weight, but it also concentrates on helping you to change your current eating habits into something that is much healthier for the whole body. If you successfully complete the HCG diet, you will be better equipped to make healthy eating choices, rather than eating the junk that you did before, and the weight should stay off even when you are done taking the HCG injections or drops.

If you end your HCG diet and go back to your old eating habits, then it is possible that you will gain weight back. If you take in too many calories for your body, this will happen no matter which diet plan you are on. However, the third phase of the HCG is meant to help you safely adjust from the weight loss portion of the HCG diet over to the maintenance phase and will make it easier for you to keep the weight off.

Approved HCG Diet Foods

You will really need to watch the foods that you are eating when you are in the second phase of the diet plan. The first phase will mostly concentrate on eating foods that you crave so you can get those temptations out of the way. The last two phases will be based off the second phase, allowing you to eat healthier than you ever imagined possible. But to see the biggest weight loss while on this diet, you need to be really mindful of what you eat during the second phase. Some of the different foods (as well as the amount of each food) you should consume during this second phase include:

Protein

You need to have one serving of protein two times each day. Each serving will be about 100 grams (3.5ounces) for each serving. You need to weigh the protein raw and make sure that no seasoning or other preparation has been done before you weigh. Some of the different protein sources that you can choose include:

- Chicken breast
- Beef (make sure that you can get this as lean as possible.
- Shrimp
- Crab
- Lobster
- White fish including tilapia, sole, sea bass, flounder, trout, cod, and catfish.
- One egg and three egg whites
- 100 grams of cottage cheese

Vegetables

You also need to take in some vegetables to provide you with the nutrients that the body requires to stay healthy. The servicing size is not indicated on this diet plan. The original protocol does not outline how big serving needs to be or how many servings you should stick with. You can eat these to satisfaction. Some vegetables that are allowed in this diet plan include:

- Tomatoes
- Spinach
- Radishes
- Onions
- Lettuce
- Fennel
- Cucumber
- Celery
- Cabbage
- Beet greens
- Asparagus

Fruits

Some of the fruits that you can enjoy on this diet plan include a handful of strawberries, one orange, half a grapefruit, and one apple

Carbs

There are a few carbs that you are allowed to have in the second phase of the HCG diet. However, most carbs are reduced because they are just so high in calories. The carbs that you are allowed to have include one piece of Melba toast and one Grissini stick without the oil in it.

Other options

Some of the other options that you can choose from include one lemon and some milk each day. Spices and herbs are fine as long as you read the label and make sure that there aren't any fillers, sweeteners, sugars, or other things found inside of them. You should also be cautious of using sweeteners at all on this diet plan, don't consume sugar when you don't need to.

As you can see, there are some limitations that occur when you are following this diet plan. You are only allowed to have 500 calories each day on this diet plan to see the results, and you must choose from the options that are listed above. This can make it hard for some people who are just getting started, but if you really want to see results with this diet plan, you will need to stick to the limitations.

Easy HCG Diet Recipes

One of the hardest things that you will need to figure out with the HCG diet is what foods you are allowed to eat. You are only allowed to have up to 500 calories in a whole day, and you can quickly go through these if you are not careful. Not only do you want to stick with the right amount of calories, but you also want to make sure that you are getting foods that will fill you up as much as possible and won't make you feel deprived at the end of the day.

This chapter will provide you with some of the best recipes that you can enjoy on the HCG diet. They are full of healthy and lean meats, good fruits and vegetables, and the limited carbs that you are allowed to have on the HCG diet. So, take a look through these recipes, as well as the meal plan in the next chapter, to help you get started with this diet today.

Clarifications:

c = cup (1 cup is 236ml)
Tsp = teaspoon (1 teaspoon is 5ml)
Tbsp = tablespoon (1 tablespoon is 15ml)
O = ounce (1 ounce is 28grams)

Breakfast Recipes

Easy Coleslaw

What's in it

- Salt
- Cumin
- Rosemary
- Basil
- Vinegar (.25 c.)
- Shredded cabbage (3.5 o.)

How's it done

1. Take out a big bowl and mix the vinegar and cabbage.
2. Season with the cumin, salt, rosemary, and basil. Stir around and then serve when ready.

Apple Salad

What's in it

- Apple cider vinegar (2 Tbsp.)
- Water (1 Tbsp.)
- Chopped apple (.5)
- Sliced cucumber (1)
- Pepper
- Garlic salt

How's it done

1. Take out a bowl and combine the apple and cucumber together.
2. Inside a Mason jar, shake together the garlic salt, pepper, water, and apple cider vinegar. Shake around to combine.
3. Pour this dressing over the salad and serve.

Garlic Greens

What's in it

- Salt
- Lemon juice (4 Tbsp.)
- Chopped onion (2 Tbsp.)
- Red pepper flakes (.25 tsp.)
- Minced garlic cloves (3)
- Vegetable broth (.25 c.)
- Greens of your choice (2 c.)

How's it done

1. Bring the broth (or you can substitute in water if you would like) to boil in a pot. Add the spices, onion, and garlic to the pot as well.
2. After the mixture is boiling, add the greens and then cook with the lid on the pot for the next fifteen minutes.
3. Season with the salt and lemon and then taste.

Lemon Spinach Soup

What's in it

- Salt
- Thyme (.5 tsp.)
- Spinach (1 lb.)
- Lemon juice (2 tsp.)
- Vegetable broth (2 c.)

How's it done

1. Put the salt, thyme, broth, and lemon juice into a pot. Allow all of the ingredients to come to a boil.
2. Add your spinach to the bottom of a few bowls and then pour the boiling ingredients on top before serving.

Asparagus Soup

What's in it

- Chicken broth (.25 c.)
- Asparagus (.25 lb.)
- Salt
- Pepper
- Garlic powder (.25 tsp.)

How's it done

1. Add all of the ingredients into a pot and let them cook until your vegetables are tender.
2. When this is done, add all the ingredients in a blender. Blend to make smooth and then serve.

Creole Cucumbers

What's in it

- Creole seasoning (.25 tsp.)
- Sliced cucumbers (2 c.)

How's it done

1. Toss the cucumbers and the seasoning together until well combined and then serve.

Caramelized Onions

What's in it

- Water (6 Tbsp.)
- Pepper
- Salt
- Sliced sweet onion (1)

How's it done

2. Heat up your frying pan on the stove. Add the onions in and season to your personal tastes.
3. Let the onions cook until they start to brown. At this time, add in the water, going one tablespoon at a time. go until the water evaporates completely.
4. Serve these warm.

Lemon Asparagus

What's in it

- Salt
- Pepper
- Lemon juice (1 Tbsp.)
- Asparagus (.33 lb.)

How's it done

1. Take out a pot and fill it halfway with water. Bring this water to a boil.
2. Rinse and then dry your asparagus, taking the time to break off the tough part of the stem. Cut the remaining part into one-inch pieces.
3. Drop the asparagus into the boiling water. Reduce to a simmer and cook for a few minutes.
4. After this time is done, drain out the water. Toss with the lemon juice, pepper, and salt.

Onion Rings

What's in it

- Pepper
- Salt
- Cayenne pepper (.25 tsp.)
- Skim milk (1 Tbsp.)
- Crumbled melba toast
- Onion, sliced into rings (.5)

How's it done

1. Allow the oven some time to heat up to 350 degrees. While that is heating up, mix the milk with the salt and the cayenne pepper.
2. Dip your onion rings into this mixture before adding to the melba toast crumbs. Lay these out on a baking sheet and place into the oven.
3. Allow these to bake for a few minutes. After seven minutes have passed, flip the onion rings around and bake for an additional seven minutes. Serve warm.

Spiced Apples

What's in it

- Allspice (.25 tsp.)
- Cinnamon (.5 tsp.)
- Apple, cubed (1)

How's it done

1. Place all of the ingredients together in a bowl and then place the bowl into the microwave.
2. Let this bake for a minute and a half in the microwave and then serve warm.

Candy Apples

What's in it

- Stevia (4 packets)
- Apples (4)
- Water (2 c.)
- Vanilla (1 tsp.)
- Cinnamon (1 tsp.)

How's it done

1. Allow the oven to heat up to 350 degrees. Take out a baking dish and add the apples inside with the water.
2. Sprinkle the cinnamon and the stevia on the apples before adding to the oven.
3. After an hour, you can take the apples out of the oven. Mix the vanilla into the water and then pour this over the apples before serving.

Strawberry Orange Smoothie

What's in it

- Stevia (.5 tsp.)
- Ice (.75 c.)
- Orange juice (.33 c.)
- Strawberries (1 c.)

How's it done

1. Add the stevia, ice, orange juice, and strawberries into the blender. Add the lid on top.
2. Blend the ingredients until they are smooth.

Strawberry Shortcake

What's in it

- Vanilla crème stevia (2 drops)
- Melba toast (1)
- Sliced strawberry (1)

How's it done

1. Take the toast out and lay it on your plate.
2. Place the strawberry on the toast before adding the stevia. Serve right away.

Lunch Recipes

Steak Fajitas

What's in it

- Lime juice (2 Tbsp.)
- Sliced onion (1)
- Green pepper, sliced (1)
- Round steak (3.5)
- Water (.25 c.)
- Garlic powder (.25 tsp.)
- Onion powder (.5 tsp.)
- Cumin (.5 tsp.)
- Salt (1 tsp.)

How's it done

1. Take out a plastic bag and mix the water and the spices together inside.
2. Add the pepper, onion, and steak. Seal up the bag, making sure to press most of the air out of the bag.
3. Knead the bag a big to make sure that the ingredients are all combined. Leave in the fridge for an additional 20 minutes.
4. Heat up a frying pan and then add in the contents from your plastic bag. Cook so the steak is completely done, and the vegetables are soft.
5. Serve this warm.

Tomato Burger

What's in it

- Lettuce leaf (1)
- Coriander
- Dill (.25 tsp.)
- Pepper
- Salt
- Onion powder (1 pinch)
- Garlic powder (1 pinch)
- Tomato slices (2)
- Ground beef (3.5 oz.)

How's it done

1. Mix the beef with the spices and then make into a patty.
2. Preheat the grill before adding the patty to the grill. Cook it until the patty reaches the desired doneness.
3. Place the patty between two slices of tomato and the lettuce before serving.

Veal Chops

What's in it

1. Pepper
2. Salt
3. Lemon juice (.5 Tbsp.)
4. Veal chops (3.5 oz.)

How's it done

- Add the lemon juice and the veal to a plastic bag. Let these marinate together for about an hour.
- After that time is up, heat up a frying pan and then season the veal with the pepper and salt. Add the veal to the pan and let it cook for a bit on each side.
- Squeeze on some more lemon juice over the meat and then serve.

Taco Salad

What's in it

- Chopped tomato (1)
- Melba toast, chopped up
- Pepper
- Salt
- Minced cilantro (1 Tbsp.)
- Cooked ground beef (3.5 oz.)
- Sliced lettuce (2 c.)

How's it done

1. Take out a big salad bowl. Toss together all of the ingredients and then serve right away.

Onions and Citrus Beef

What's in it

- Sliced onion (3.5 o.)
- Juice from half a lemon
- Beef (3.5 oz.)

How's it done

2. Bring out a pan and add the pepper and salt to it. Then add the onions with some water. Simmer these ingredients together for three minutes.
3. At this time, add the lemon juice and the meat. Cook the meat until it reaches the desired doneness.
4. Serve warm with the pan juices.

Beef Chili

What's in it

- Oregano (1 pinch)
- Chili powder (.25 tsp.)
- Onion powder (1 pinch)
- Garlic powder (1 pinch)
- Crushed garlic cloves (2)
- Minced onion (1 Tbsp.)
- Water (.5 c.)
- Chopped tomatoes (1 c.)
- Ground beef (3.5 oz.)
- Pepper
- Salt
- Cayenne pepper

How's it done

1. Take out a small skillet and brown the beef. When the beef is done, add the tomatoes, water, garlic, and onions.
2. Add the spices as well and then simmer all of these ingredients together until the sauce has thickened.
3. Add some pepper and salt to taste and then serve with some tomato slices.

Lemon and Garlic Steaks

What's in it

- Pepper
- Salt
- Juiced and zested lemon (1)
- Minced garlic clove (1)
- Cubed steak (3.5 oz.)

How's it done

1. Heat up your frying pan. While that is heating, season the steak with your salt and pepper.
2. Add the steak to the pan and let it brown evenly. After about five minutes, add the garlic and cook a bit longer.
3. Before serving, add the lemon juice and zest. Serve the steak covered in the juices.

Chicken Fajitas

What's in it

- Salt (1 tsp.)
- Lime juice (2 Tbsp.)
- Sliced onion (1)
- Sliced green bell pepper (1)
- Sliced chicken breast (6 oz.)
- Water (.25 c.)
- Garlic powder (.25 tsp.)
- Onion powder (.5 tsp.)
- Cumin (.5 tsp.)

How's it done

1. Take out a plastic bag and mix the water and spices together inside.
2. Add the pepper, onion, and chicken and seal the bag, making sure to get rid of most of the air.
3. Knead the ingredients around a bit to ensure that they are covered and then let it set in the fridge for another 20 minutes.
4. After this time, heat up a frying pan and add in all the ingredients. Let the chicken cook completely, making sure to stir the whole time. Serve warm.

Orange Chicken

What's in it

- Sliced orange (1)
- Cooked broccoli (3.5 oz.)
- Chicken (3.5 oz.)
- Hot water (.25 c.)
- Chai tea bag (1)

How's it done

1. To start this recipe, steep a tea bag in the hot water in a pan. You will need to do this for about three minutes.
2. After this time, take the tea bag out of the water. Add the chicken pieces and let them simmer in the water until completely cooked.
3. Toss the chicken together with the rest of the tea, the oranges, and the broccoli. Season the way that you would like and enjoy.

Cucumber Shrimp Salad

What's in it

- Hot sauce, sugar-free
- Lemon (.5)
- White vinegar
- Sliced cucumbers (1 c.)
- Diced shrimp (125 grams)

How's it done

1. Take the shrimp and cook it by steaming or boiling. When these are done, add the hot sauce to the shrimp and allow them to cool down in the fridge for an hour.
2. When the shrimp is ready, add it to a bowl with the lemon, white vinegar, and cucumber. Serve with some melba toast before enjoying.

Veggie Salad

What's in it

- Greens (1 c.)
- Spinach (1 c.)
- Chopped turkey (100 oz.)
- Red pepper flakes (.5 tsp.)
- Pepper (.5 tsp.)
- Lemon (.5)
- Chopped cucumber (.5 c.)
- Chopped onion (.5 c.)

How's it done

1. Take out a big salad bowl and add all of the vegetables together. Top this with the turkey.
2. Add the lemon juice on top like a dressing and then season with the rest of the ingredients. Serve right away.

Crab Salad

What's in it

- Romaine lettuce (2 c.)
- Melba rounds
- Crab meat (100 grams)
- *Honey mustard dressing*
- Onion powder (.5 tsp.)
- Garlic powder (.5 tsp.)
- Pepper (.5 tsp.)
- Salt (.5 tsp.)
- Brown mustard, no sugar (2.5 Tbsp.)
- Stevia (1 c.) mixed with water (1 c.)

How's it done

1. To make the dressing, place all the ingredients into a jar and shake until well combined. Place into a container that is airtight and then leave in the fridge until ready to use.
2. To work on the salad, you can combine the romaine lettuce with the crab meat in a bowl.
3. Top with a few tablespoons of the honey mustard dressing and serve with a few melba rounds to enjoy.

Dinner Recipes

Lemon Basil Chicken

What's in it

- Chopped tomatoes (3.5 oz.)
- Chicken (3.5 oz.)
- Basil
- Juice from a lemon (.5)

How's it done

1. Add the chicken to a frying pan along with the lemon juice and a bit more water if needed.
2. Cook this on a medium heat setting for about four minutes.
3. After this time, add the basil and the tomatoes before turning the heat down to low.
4. Simmer the chicken until it is completely cooked. Serve this over some lettuce and enjoy.

Chicken and Cabbage Wraps

What's in it

- Grated ginger (1 Tbsp.)
- Pepper (.25 Tbsp.)
- Salt (.25 Tbsp.)
- Onion powder (.25 tsp.)
- Balsamic vinegar (3 Tbsp.)
- Minced garlic clove (1)
- Red cabbage leaves (2)
- Chicken (3.5 oz.)

How's it done

1. To start this recipe, mix together the pepper, vinegar, onion powder, salt, garlic, and ginger.
2. Toss the chicken in with this mixture and then cook on the stove with a medium-high heat until it is cooked through.
3. Add in the cabbage leaves at this time and heat to make them soft. But, you don't want them cooked much.
4. Lay the cabbage leaves out and place half the chicken mix on each one. Roll them up tightly before serving.

Basil Chicken

What's in it

- Hot pepper sauce (.25 tsp.)
- Salt (.5 tsp.)
- Minced basil (.25 c.)
- Chicken breast, sliced (2 c.)
- Chopped tomatoes (2.5 c.)
- Minced garlic (1)
- Chopped onion (.5 c.)
- Cooking spray

How's it done

1. Take out a frying pan and prepare it with some cooking spray. Heat up some garlic and onions in the frying pan.
2. When the onions and garlic are done, add in the chicken along with the rest of the ingredients. Turn the heat down a little bit.
3. Simmer this mixture, allowing it to cook until the tomatoes are soft and the chicken is cooked through.

Blackened Chicken

What's in it

- Onion powder (.25 tsp.)
- Chicken breasts (2)
- White pepper (.25 tsp.)
- Dried thyme (.25 tsp.)
- Cumin (.25 tsp.)
- Cayenne pepper (.25 tsp.)
- Salt (.25 tsp.)
- Paprika (.5 tsp.)

How's it done

1. Allow the oven some time to heat up to 350 degrees. While the oven is heating up, prepare a cookie sheet with some cooking spray.
2. Take out a bowl and toss all of the spices together. Use the cooking spray to help oil your chicken on both sides before coating with the spices.
3. Add the chicken to the frying pan, cooking on each side for a minute. Add the chicken to the cookie sheet and then place into the oven.
4. Cook this chicken until the juices start to run clear and then serve.

Chicken Chili

What's in it

- Pepper
- Salt
- Thyme (.5 tsp.)
- Oregano (.5 tsp.)
- Chili powder (.5 tsp.)
- Cumin (.5 tsp.)
- Minced garlic cloves (2)
- Water (2 c.)
- Chopped Roma tomatoes (2)
- Grated cabbage (1 c.)
- Ground beef (3.5 oz.)

How's it done

1. Take out a frying pan and cook the garlic and the meat together until the meat is completely cooked through. Add in the spices and the water and bring it all to a boil.
2. Now add in the cabbage and cook until it becomes tender. Stir in the tomato and let it simmer for a bit longer before serving.

Chicken Adobo

What's in it

- Ginger (.25 tsp.)
- Bay leaf (1)
- Minced garlic clove (1)
- Diced onion (.25)
- Soy sauce (.25 c.)
- Apple cider vinegar (.25 c.)
- Chicken breast (1)

How's it done

1. Use some cooking spray to grease up a frying pan. Then add the garlic and onion until they are tender.
2. Add the rest of the ingredients except the chicken. Let these cook, so they start to have bubbles form.
3. Add the chicken and simmer until it is completely cooked through, which will take about ten minutes. Serve warm.

Jerk Turkey Salad

What's in it

- Sliced celery (.25 c.)
- Strawberries (2 oz.)
- Chopped pineapple (2 oz.)
- Peeled and sliced cucumber (.5)
- Caribbean jerk seasoning (1 Tbsp.)
- Turkey breast (3.5 oz.)
- Salt
- Cumin
- Lime juice (.25 c.)
- Green onion (2 slices)

How's it done

1. Take the turkey breast and season it with the jerk seasoning
2. Turn on your grill or heat up a frying pan and add the turkey to it. Cook so the turkey is completely done.
3. Take the turkey from the heat and let it have some time to cool down before slicing into small pieces.
4. Toss the turkey in with the rest of the ingredients and serve warm.

Spicy Crab

What's in it

- Lime juice (1 tsp.)
- Crab meat (3.5 oz.)
- Sliced cucumber (.5)
- Red pepper flakes
- Dry mustard powder (.5 tsp.)
- Chopped green onions (1 tsp.)
- Water (1 tsp.)

How's it done

1. Take out a bowl and mix together the crab and the spices. When those are well combined, top with the lime juice and the water.
2. Before serving, add in the cucumber slices, stir around, and then serve.

Grilled Shrimp

What's in it

- Cooked shrimp (6 oz.)
- Cumin (1 tsp.)
- Salt (1 tsp.)
- Minced garlic cloves (3)
- Juice from one lemon
- Chopped cilantro (.25 c.)

How's it done

1. To start this recipe, take all of the ingredients and toss them into a plastic bag. Place in the fridge to marinate for an hour.
2. Turn on the grill. When the grill is ready, add the shrimp on to cook.
3. The shrimp will be done when it starts to look opaque. Take off the grill and serve warm.

Seafood Gumbo

What's in it

- Stevia (1 packet)
- Cayenne pepper (.25 tsp.)
- Garlic powder (.25 tsp.)
- Creole seasoning (.25 tsp.)
- Onion salt (.25 tsp.)
- Chopped Roma tomatoes (2)
- Minced garlic clove (1)
- Seafood of choice (3.5 oz.)

How's it done

1. Take out a skillet and cook the seafood and garlic for about a minute on a high heat setting.
2. After this time, add the rest of the ingredients, taking the time to reduce the heat, so they are all simmering.
3. After fifteen minutes, the dish is ready to eat.

Fish Tacos

What's in it

- Sliced white fish (3.5 oz.)
- Melba toast
- Cabbage leaves (1 to 2 leaves)
- Pepper
- Salt
- Onion powder (1 pinch)
- Garlic powder (1 pinch)
- Chili powder (1 pinch)

How's it done

1. To start this recipe, toss together the spices and the fish into a frying pan, adding a bit of water. Cook the fish until it is done and then drain out the excess water.
2. Place the cabbage in the microwave for 30 seconds to help the leaves become soft.
3. Split up the fish mixture and add half to each leaf.
4. Sprinkle the melba toast over the fish, roll it up, and then serve.

Diet Calendar to Get You Started

When you are getting started on the HCG diet, there are a lot of things to consider. You need to keep track of all the injections that you need to take in, and you must make sure that you are sticking to the calorie content that you need. Picking out a good meal plan can seem almost impossible.

That is why we will make it easy for you. Using the recipes that are found in the last chapter, you can follow this basic meal plan that will help you out. Here we are providing you with four weeks on the HCG diet. Since the HCG diet is recommended for three to six weeks, this will at least give you a good start on the diet plan. You can then reuse some of the recipes or come up with some of your own to finish out the last few weeks if you need.

Sunday	Monday	Tuesday	Wednesday	Thursday	Friday	Saturday
	1 B: Easy Coleslaw L: Steak Fajitas D: Lemon Basil Chicken	2 B: Apple Salad L: Tomato Burger D: Chicken and Cabbage Wraps	3 B: Garlic Greens L: Veal Chops D: Basil Chicken	4 B: Lemon Spinach Soup L: Taco Salad D: Blackened Chicken	5 B: Asparagus Soup L: Onions and Citrus Beef D: Chicken Chili	6 B: Creole Cucumbers L: Beef Chili D: Chicken Adobo
7 B: Caramelized Onions L: Lemon Garlic Steaks D: Jerk Turkey Salad	8 B: Lemon Asparagus L: Chicken Fajitas D: Spicy Crab	9 B: Easy Coleslaw L: Steak Fajitas D: Chicken and Cabbage Wraps	10 B: Onion Rings L: Taco Salad D: Lemon Basil Chicken	11 B: Spiced Apples L: Beef Chili D: Blackened Chicken	12 B: Strawberry Orange Smoothie L: Orange Chicken D: Grilled Shrimp	13 B: Apple Salad L: Cucumber Shrimp Salad D: Basil Chicken
14 B: Strawberry Shortcake L: Veggie Salad D: Seafood Gumbo	15 B: Apple Salad L: Lemon Garlic Steaks D: Jerk Turkey Salad	16 B: Spiced Apples L: Chicken Fajitas D: Chicken Adobo	17 B: Candy Apples L: Tomato Burger D: Spicy Crab	18 B: Lemon Spinach Soup L: Veal Chops D: Grilled Shrimp	19 B: Strawberry Orange Smoothie L: Crab Salad D: Fish Tacos	20 B: Onion Rings L: Orange Chicken D: Chicken Chili

21	22	23	24	25	26	27
B: Strawberry Shortcake L: Veal Chops D: Basil Chicken	B: Candy Apples L: Cucumber Shrimp Salad D: Seafood Gumbo	B: Garlic Greens L: Veggie Salad D: Spicy Crab	B: Creole Cucumbers L: Crab Salad D: Lemon Basil Chicken	B: Asparagus Soup L: Beef Chili D: Blackened Chicken	B: Spiced Apples L: Onions and Citrus Beef D: Chicken Adobo	B: Lemon Spinach Soup L: Lemon Garlic Steaks D: Fish Tacos
28	29	30	31			
B: Lemon Asparagus L: Crab Salad D: Grilled Shrimp	B: Onion Rings L: Chicken Fajitas D: Jerk Turkey Salad	B: Caramelized Onions L: Taco Salad D: Chicken Chili	B: Easy Coleslaw L: Tomato Burger D: Chicken and Cabbage Wraps			

71

Conclusion

Thank you for making it through to the end of this book, let's hope it was informative and able to provide you with all of the tools you need to achieve your goals whatever they may be.

The next step is to get started on the HCG diet. This is not the easiest diet plan out there. Most people will have trouble sticking with a diet plan that keeps them limited to only 500 calories each day. Add in that you also need to take injections or drops each day, and you can see where this diet plan is not the easiest. But for those who are looking to lose some real weight quickly, the HCG diet is one of the most effective diet plans out there.

This guidebook spent some time talking about everything you need to know to get started with the HCG diet. From understanding the history of this diet plan to looking at some of the benefits and the different phases of this diet, you will learn everything that you need to be successful the first time with the HCG diet.

Finally, if you found this book useful in any way, a review on Amazon is always appreciated!

41305699R00044

Made in the USA
San Bernardino, CA
02 July 2019